HEALING

CIRCLES

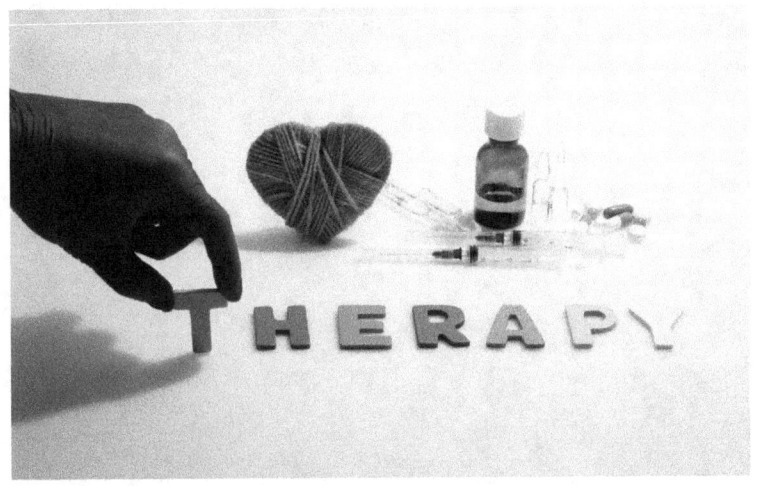

Embracing Growth and Resilience
Through Group Therapy

Curtis C. Figueroa

HEALING CIRCLES

Table of contents

INTRODUCTION

In the vast tapestry of human existence, there are threads that bind us together, unseen but potent in their ability to heal and transform. One such thread weaves through the lives of individuals seeking solace, growth, and resilience: group therapy. Welcome to "Healing Circles: Embracing Growth and Resilience Through Group Therapy," where we embark on a profound journey of self-discovery, shared experiences, and renewed hope.

Throughout history, humans have sought out connection as a means to find meaning in their struggles and triumphs. We gather around campfires, sit at communal tables, and form circles of trust. It is within these sacred spaces that we find the power of vulnerability, the strength of genuine connections, and the transformative embrace of healing.

Let me share with you a tale of courage, perseverance, and redemption, a story that embodies the essence of what lies within these pages—a tale of Sara, a woman who had weathered life's harshest storms but emerged from the tempest stronger than ever.

Sara's Story: A Journey to Healing

Once, Sara was a vibrant soul, dancing through life with exuberance. Yet, like all of us, her life took an unexpected turn—a cruel twist of fate that left her heart shattered into a million pieces. A sudden loss tore her world asunder, leaving her drowning in a sea of grief and despair.

HEALING CIRCLES

Despite her loved ones' best intentions, Sara found herself struggling to resurface, to find solid ground once more. Her heartache seemed insurmountable, an unscalable mountain casting an unyielding shadow over her life.

Then, one day, fate led her to a small gathering of individuals with similar scars, where she hesitantly stepped into the circle of Healing Circles—a group therapy session unlike any other. At first, Sara felt unsure, the weight of her grief pressing against her chest, suffocating her. But within those warm, accepting eyes and empathetic smiles, she found a glimmer of hope.

As she began to share her story, piece by broken piece, something magical began to happen. The walls she had erected around her heart began to crumble. In the embrace of these kindred souls, she discovered the liberating power of vulnerability—a gift that bound them together in a tapestry of shared understanding.

With each passing session, Sara found herself not only speaking but truly being heard. Her pain was acknowledged, her grief validated, and her resilience celebrated. The group became her refuge, where she could shed the armor she had worn for far too long and, for the first time, allow herself to heal.

As weeks turned into months, Sara noticed a remarkable transformation within herself. The healing she had yearned for had begun. Empowered by the wisdom and support of her peers, she learned to navigate life's tumultuous waters with newfound resilience. Through the power of connection and collective strength, she embraced her vulnerability and, in turn, discovered her hidden wellspring of courage.

HEALING CIRCLES

And so, the tale of Sara illustrates the transformative magic that lies within the realm of group therapy—a haven of shared growth, where individuals find the courage to confront their pain and forge ahead with newfound purpose.

Dear reader, within these pages, you will find not only Sara's story but the stories of countless others whose lives have been irrevocably touched by the power of Healing Circles. As we delve into the intricacies of group therapy, we invite you to embark on a journey of self-exploration, personal breakthroughs, and the radiant embrace of resilience.

Together, we shall uncover the secrets of creating a safe and supportive environment, harnessing the strength of diversity, and

HEALING CIRCLES

cultivating the art of active listening. In "Healing Circles," you will discover the tools to rebuild and renew, to embrace vulnerability as a strength, and to emerge stronger than ever before.

—CHAPTER ONE—

The Power of Shared Healing

In the opening chapter of "Healing Circles," we delve into the very essence of group therapy—the undeniable power of shared healing. At the heart of this concept lies the understanding that individuals are not alone in their struggles. When they gather within a supportive community, a profound sense of validation, empathy, and understanding washes over them, gently dissolving the barriers that isolate and alienate.

Consider the story of Mark, a combat veteran haunted by the ghosts of war. Plagued by memories he could neither escape nor articulate, he withdrew from the world, believing his pain was incomprehensible to others.

But within the crucible of a veterans' support group, Mark discovered a kinship that transcended words. Surrounded by fellow warriors who had traversed similar emotional battlegrounds, he found solace in shared experiences.

In the sanctuary of understanding, the weight of his pain began to lift, and hope found its way back into his heart.

1.1 Emphasizes the transformational potential of group therapy

The ability to transcend loneliness and find validation in the eyes of others who have weathered similar storms.

As we explore the stories of individuals like Mark, we witness the gradual metamorphosis from isolation to connection—a metamorphosis that ignites a shared journey toward healing.

1.2 Understanding Group Therapy

In the pursuit of healing, it becomes vital to comprehend the fundamental principles and workings of group therapy. In 1.2, we shed light on the mechanics that drive Healing Circles forward.

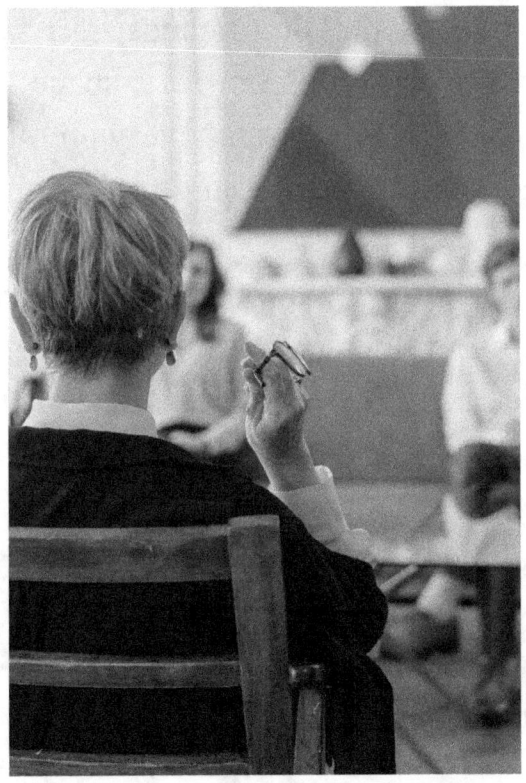

Meet Sarah, a young woman navigating the challenges of anxiety and self-doubt.

HEALING CIRCLES

As she hesitantly joined a women's empowerment group, Sarah found herself intrigued by the structure and dynamics at play. Led by a skilled therapist, the group encouraged open dialogue, active listening, and non-judgmental feedback. Through this, Sarah grasped the significance of a safe and supportive environment—a space where every voice resonated and every emotion was met with compassionate understanding.

1.2 underscores the importance of an expertly guided group therapy setting, where a skilled therapist acts as a compassionate facilitator, steering the sessions toward growth and healing. The chapter emphasizes the establishment of trust, confidentiality, and shared goals, setting the stage for transformative experiences that redefine the participants' perception of therapy itself.

Together, 1.1 and 1.2 lay the foundation for the transformative journey that awaits within "Healing Circles." By exploring the power of shared healing and understanding the essential elements that drive group therapy, readers are primed to embark on a voyage of resilience, discovery, and communal strength that transcends individual boundaries.

–CHAPTER TWO–

The Foundation of Healing Circles

Chapter 2 of "Healing Circles" delves into the core principles that form the foundation of these transformative therapeutic communities.

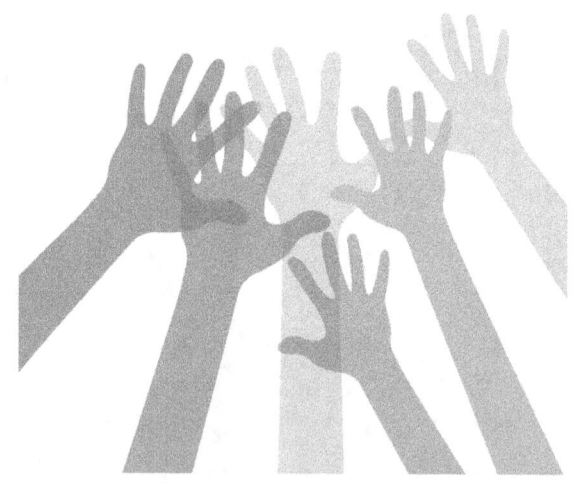

In the sacred space of Healing Circles, participants find themselves gently cradled by a supportive environment, fostering a sense of trust, vulnerability, and emotional safety.

This chapter unravels the essential building blocks that create such an environment, where healing becomes not only possible but also profound.

2.1 Creating a Safe and Supportive Environment

The cornerstone of Healing Circles lies in the creation of a safe and supportive environment—one where individuals feel seen, heard, and accepted unconditionally. In this chapter, we explore how skilled therapists and facilitators craft this nurturing space, establishing ground rules that prioritize respect, confidentiality, and compassion. Through the art of active listening and empathetic understanding, participants experience a unique sense of belonging, free from judgment and criticism.

Imagine Jennifer, a survivor of emotional abuse who believed her voice was insignificant. Cautiously entering a Healing Circle for survivors of trauma, she discovered a refuge in which her words were met with empathy and validation. The therapeutic cocoon provided by the group allowed her to gradually reclaim her sense of self-worth and recognize her inherent strength.

2.2 Establishing Trust and Confidentiality

Trust is the lifeblood of Healing Circles, flowing through every interaction, binding individuals together in an unbreakable bond. In chapter 2.2, we explore the delicate process of building trust among group members and the vital role that confidentiality plays in fostering an environment where individuals feel secure in sharing their deepest vulnerabilities.

Consider Daniel, a man grappling with addiction, who found himself hesitant to open up during his first group therapy session. However, as he witnessed the unwavering support and confidentiality upheld by his peers, he began to feel a newfound sense of safety. In time, Daniel felt empowered to confront his struggles head-on, knowing that his fellow participants were his steadfast allies on the path to recovery.

2.3 Setting Goals and Expectations

Every Healing Circle begins with a collective agreement to set shared goals and expectations. Chapter 2.3 delves into the collaborative process that participants undertake to establish the purpose and trajectory of their therapeutic journey. This mutual commitment cultivates a sense of responsibility and motivation within the group, uniting individuals in their pursuit of growth and healing.

Imagine a grief support group where each participant shares their unique aspirations—to find closure, to honor their loved ones' memories, or to develop coping mechanisms. As they embark on this shared odyssey, they find inspiration and accountability in each other's aspirations, propelling their healing process forward.

Conclusion:

Within the foundation of Healing Circles lie the seeds of transformation, watered by trust, nurtured by confidentiality, and guided by collective purpose. As we explore the elements that underpin these transformative therapeutic communities, we begin to understand the profound impact they have on participants' lives. In the safe and supportive haven of Healing Circles, individuals embark on a journey of self-discovery, resilience, and growth, their hearts intertwined as they walk together toward the light of healing.

–CHAPTER THREE–

The Journey of Vulnerability

Chapter 3 of "Healing Circles" explores the profound and transformative power of vulnerability—the essence of baring one's soul in the presence of others. In a world often marked by a relentless pursuit of strength and stoicism, the act of embracing vulnerability can be seen as an act of courage. This chapter delves into how Healing Circles create a nurturing space where vulnerability is not only accepted but celebrated as a stepping stone to healing.

3.1 Embracing Vulnerability as a Strength

In today's fast-paced and competitive world, vulnerability is often misconstrued as weakness. However, Healing Circles offer a different perspective—one that cherishes vulnerability as a profound strength. As the world faces unprecedented challenges and uncertainties, acknowledging vulnerability becomes more critical than ever.

In the context of current global situations, such as the aftermath of a pandemic, economic instability, and the emotional toll of prolonged isolation, individuals find themselves navigating a labyrinth of emotions. The journey of embracing vulnerability within Healing Circles becomes a beacon of hope, reminding participants that it is okay to seek support, to express fears and insecurities, and to lean on others during times of hardship.

3.2 Overcoming Fear of Judgment

One of the barriers to vulnerability is the fear of judgment—a belief that exposing one's innermost struggles will lead to rejection or criticism. Chapter 3.2 explores how Healing Circles dismantle this fear by fostering an environment of empathy and compassion. As individuals witness their peers sharing their vulnerabilities without fear of reproach, they begin to perceive vulnerability as an act of bravery rather than weakness.

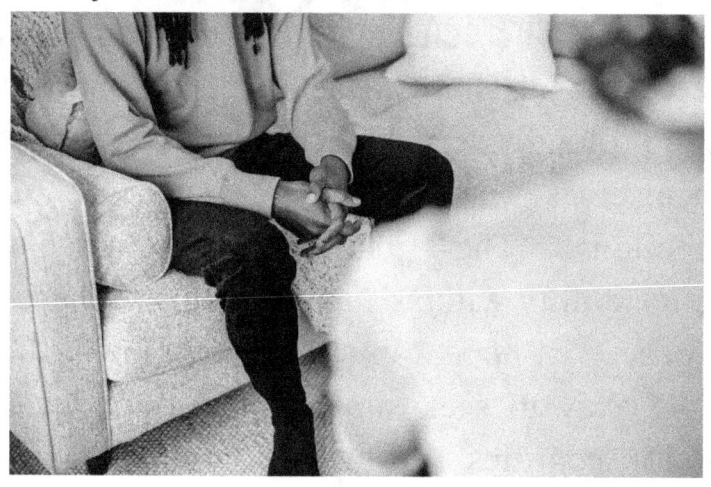

In the broader context of the current world situation, where divisions and prejudices have at times overshadowed the collective sense of humanity, Healing Circles offer a refuge of acceptance and understanding. These circles demonstrate that when judgment is replaced by compassion, individuals feel empowered to confront their challenges head-on and find healing in shared experiences.

3.3 Unveiling Hidden Emotions

In Healing Circles, participants are encouraged to explore the depth of their emotions—to unveil hidden wounds that might have remained buried for years. The therapeutic power of emotional expression creates profound connections among participants, paving the way for collective healing.

Amidst the myriad of emotions stirred by the current world situation, from anxiety and grief to hope and resilience, Healing Circles provide an outlet for individuals to process and navigate their feelings. By unveiling hidden emotions, participants learn to embrace their vulnerabilities, paving the way for transformative growth and resilience.

Conclusion:

Chapter 3 of "Healing Circles" shines a spotlight on the transformative journey of vulnerability. In the current world situation, where the human experience has been marked by uncertainty and division, the principles of Healing Circles resonate deeply. By embracing vulnerability as a strength, overcoming the fear of judgment, and unveiling hidden emotions, participants find a sanctuary to heal and connect with one another. In the embrace of shared vulnerability, Healing Circles illuminate a path toward collective healing and empowerment, reminding us that in acknowledging our humanity and supporting one another, we cultivate a resilient and compassionate world.

–CHAPTER FOUR–

The Healing Power of Connection

In the intricate tapestry of human existence, connection forms the threads that bind us together, weaving a fabric of shared experiences and emotions. Chapter 4 of "Healing Circles" delves into the profound healing power of connection, illuminating how the bonds forged within these therapeutic communities become a catalyst for transformation and growth.

4.1 Forming Genuine Bonds with Others

At the heart of Healing Circles lies the potent magic of genuine connections. In these intimate settings, participants transcend the surface level of acquaintance, forging deep and authentic bonds with one another. As they share their stories, fears, and triumphs, they recognize the universality of human experience—a reminder that we all navigate the labyrinth of life with its joys and sorrows.

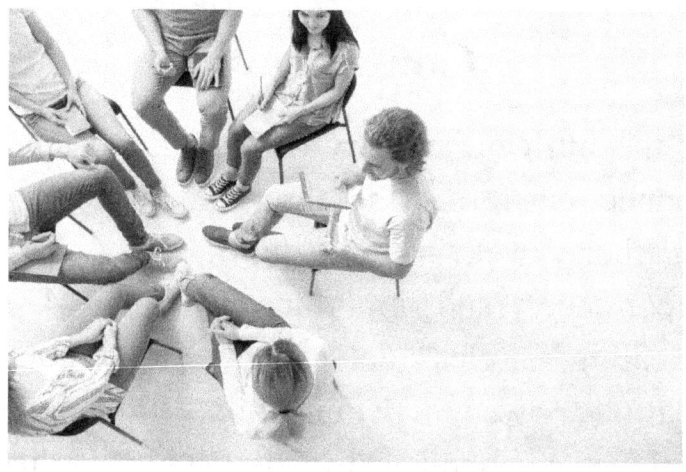

In the current era, where technology has both connected and distanced us, genuine human connections have become increasingly vital. Healing Circles act as a sanctuary in which individuals can rekindle their innate need for human interaction, providing an antidote to the isolation that modernity sometimes bestows upon us.

4.2 Empathy and Compassion in Group Therapy

Empathy and compassion are the lifeblood of Healing Circles, flowing freely among participants. Chapter 4.2 explores how these essential virtues act as conduits for healing. In the compassionate embrace of fellow participants, individuals feel seen, heard, and understood, creating a space where emotional wounds can be tended to and hearts can be mended.

In a world often fraught with divisiveness and conflict, Healing Circles stand as beacons of compassion, reminding us of our shared humanity. Empathy flourishes within these circles, dissolving barriers and fostering a sense of unity. As participants extend empathy to one another, they learn to cultivate it within themselves, creating a ripple effect that extends far beyond the bounds of the group therapy setting.

4.3 Building a Sense of Belonging

In Healing Circles, the intangible feeling of belonging takes root, anchoring participants to a community that supports, uplifts, and understands them unconditionally. Chapter 4.3 delves into how this sense of belonging becomes a nurturing cocoon, allowing individuals to shed their emotional armor and reveal their true selves.

In a world where feelings of alienation and disconnection are all too prevalent, the Healing Circles experience stands as a testament to the power of belonging. As individuals bond over shared struggles and triumphs, they find solace in the knowledge that they are not alone on their respective journeys. The shared sense of belonging fosters a deep trust, empowering participants to explore their vulnerabilities and confront their deepest traumas.

Conclusion:

Chapter 4, "The Healing Power of Connection," unveils the profound impact of genuine bonds, empathy, and a sense of belonging within Healing Circles. In an increasingly fragmented world, these therapeutic communities serve as a testament to the innate human desire for connection and understanding. As participants embrace the healing power of connection, they become part of a transformative journey that not only mends individual hearts but also weaves a tapestry of collective healing and resilience. In the realm of Healing Circles, genuine connections bloom, compassion thrives, and the profound beauty of shared humanity blossoms into a force that transcends the boundaries of time and space.

–CHAPTER FIVE–

Transforming Pain into Purpose

In chapter 5 of "Healing Circles," we embark on a journey of profound metamorphosis—a journey that empowers individuals to transform their pain into purpose. Within the therapeutic embrace of these circles, participants confront their deepest wounds and emerge with a renewed sense of meaning and direction.

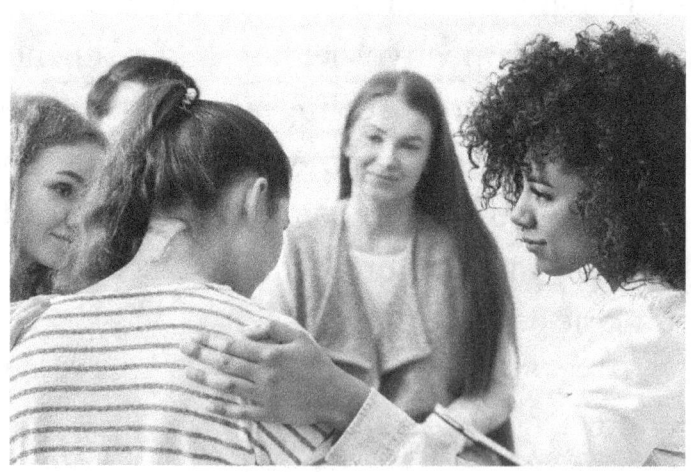

5.1 Processing Trauma and Grief Together

Healing Circles serve as a crucible for processing trauma and grief, providing participants with the opportunity to share their burdens and heal collectively. As individuals confront the raw wounds left by life's most profound challenges, they are met with unwavering support and understanding from their peers.

In the current global landscape, marked by tumultuous events and widespread loss, Healing Circles stand as an oasis for collective healing.

From the aftermath of natural disasters to the aftermath of a global pandemic, individuals find solace within these circles, knowing that their pain is not isolated, and their experiences are honored with compassion.

5.2 Finding Meaning in Adversity

Within the nurturing environment of Healing Circles, participants embark on a search for meaning in the face of adversity. Chapter 5.2 delves into the transformative process of discovering purpose amidst life's trials and tribulations. As individuals share their stories, perspectives intertwine, illuminating fresh insights and illuminating the path towards a deeper understanding of their experiences.

In the context of a world grappling with unprecedented challenges, finding meaning in adversity becomes a potent source of resilience.

Healing Circles act as a crucible, enabling participants to draw strength from their collective experiences, turning adversity into a catalyst for personal growth and a deeper connection to the human experience.

5.3 Using Challenges as Catalysts for Growth

Healing Circles empower participants to perceive challenges as opportunities for growth. Chapter 5.3 explores the art of resilience, revealing how individuals emerge from these circles with newfound strength and wisdom. As they exchange stories of transformation, participants recognize that their struggles have forged them into more resilient and compassionate beings.

In the midst of a rapidly changing world, where uncertainties abound, the ability to view challenges as catalysts for growth becomes an invaluable life skill. Within Healing Circles, participants learn to embrace change with courage and to view life's adversities as stepping stones rather than stumbling blocks.

Conclusion:

Chapter 5, "Transforming Pain into Purpose," illuminates the transformative journey that unfolds within Healing Circles. In the midst of life's most formidable trials, these therapeutic communities serve as sanctuaries of collective healing, enabling participants to process trauma and grief together. Through shared experiences, they discover profound meaning in adversity and emerge with newfound resilience and purpose.

As individuals embrace the transformative potential hidden within their pain, they become beacons of hope in an ever-changing world. Within the realm of Healing Circles, they learn to transcend their struggles, infusing their lives with purpose and embracing growth as an indomitable force that guides them towards a brighter future. In

HEALING CIRCLES

this sanctuary of healing, pain is transformed, and purpose is forged, birthing a journey of transformation that leaves no heart untouched.

–CHAPTER SIX–

Guided by Experts, Empowered by Peers

Chapter 6 of "Healing Circles" unveils the harmonious dance between expert guidance and peer support—the delicate balance that fosters a transformative and empowering therapeutic experience.

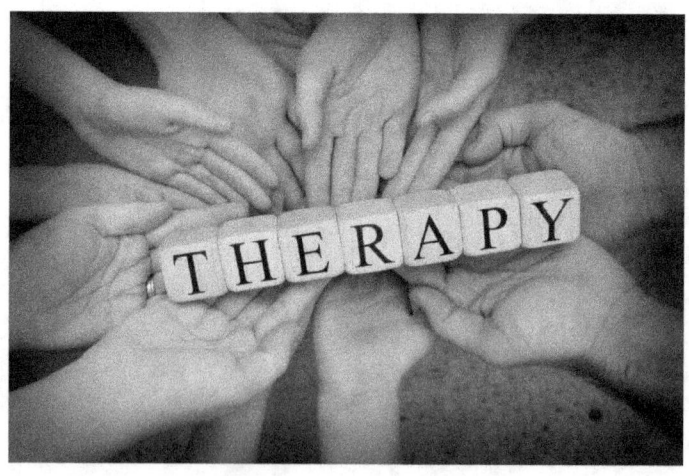

Within this chapter, we explore the unique roles of therapists and participants, understanding how their collaboration sparks profound growth and healing within the group.

6.1 The Role of Group Therapists

At the helm of Healing Circles, skilled therapists assume a crucial role as compassionate facilitators. Chapter 6.1 delves into the expertise and guidance these professionals bring to the group, orchestrating sessions with a delicate touch that allows individuals to explore their emotions and experiences in a safe and structured manner.

Therapists offer their wisdom, insight, and years of experience, providing valuable tools and techniques to navigate the labyrinth of emotions. Their expertise extends beyond providing answers; they act as guides who gently encourage self-discovery and empowerment among participants.

In the broader context of a constantly evolving world, the role of therapists within Healing Circles remains instrumental. As individuals navigate the complexities of life, they benefit from the therapeutic sanctuary created by these skilled professionals—finding solace, growth, and the strength to face life's challenges with newfound resilience.

6.2 Harnessing Collective Wisdom

Chapter 6.2 celebrates the power of collective wisdom—the innate strength found when individuals come together in mutual support and understanding. In Healing Circles, participants become sources of inspiration and encouragement for one another, collectively weaving a tapestry of shared experiences and insights.

As they share their stories, participants discover that their struggles are not unique. This realization ignites a profound sense of validation, transforming individual pain into collective healing. The diversity of perspectives within the group enriches the therapeutic experience, fostering empathy and broadening each individual's understanding of the human experience.

In the current world climate, where challenges can be overwhelming and daunting, the harnessing of collective wisdom becomes ever more crucial. Healing Circles serve as microcosms of unity, where individuals discover the immeasurable strength that emerges when people come together to support and uplift one another.

6.3 Peer Support and Validation

Central to Healing Circles is the empowering principle of peer support. Chapter 6.3 delves into how this support network becomes a source of validation and empowerment for participants. As individuals find encouragement and understanding from their peers, they begin to shed feelings of isolation, embracing the power of shared healing.

In the current global context, where feelings of disconnection and division have sometimes pervaded, Healing Circles serve as beacons of unity. Participants realize that, through the unwavering support of their peers, they can confront challenges with a newfound sense of determination.

Conclusion:

Chapter 6, "Guided by Experts, Empowered by Peers," sheds light on the symphony of expert guidance and peer support within

HEALING CIRCLES

Healing Circles. The skilled therapists act as compassionate facilitators, guiding participants on their transformative journeys, while the collective wisdom of the group empowers individuals to find strength and validation in shared experiences.

In a world that often accentuates isolation and individualism, Healing Circles serve as transformative microcosms that celebrate human connection, resilience, and unity. The collaboration between therapists and participants creates a therapeutic sanctuary, where expert guidance and peer support intertwine to weave a tapestry of healing, growth, and empowerment. Within this realm, individuals discover that they are not alone in their struggles, and the collective strength becomes a beacon of hope, guiding them towards a brighter and more compassionate world.

–CHAPTER SEVEN–

Embracing Diversity, Fostering Empathy

Chapter 7 of "Healing Circles" explores the vital principles of embracing diversity and fostering empathy within therapeutic communities. In these circles, participants from diverse backgrounds, cultures, and experiences come together to form a tapestry of humanity. This chapter delves into the transformative power of understanding and embracing differences, particularly in the context of the current world situation.

7.1 Cultivating Understanding in a Diverse Group

In Healing Circles, diversity becomes a wellspring of strength and growth. Chapter 7.1 highlights the importance of cultivating understanding and open-mindedness as participants encounter varied perspectives and life experiences within the group. The diverse amalgamation of backgrounds enriches the healing process, offering new insights and challenging preconceived notions.

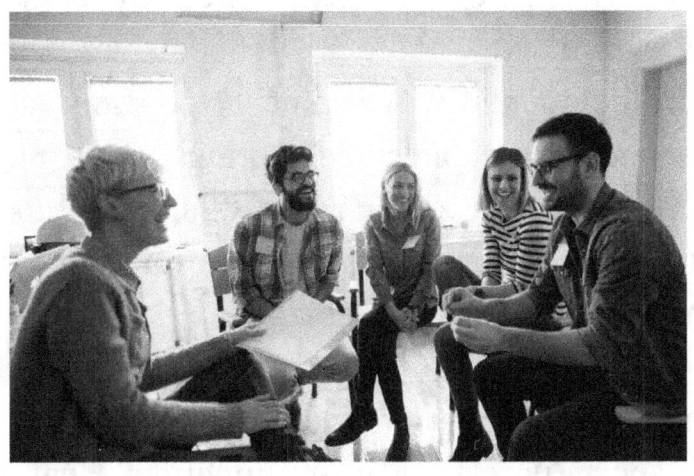

In today's interconnected global landscape, the encounters with diverse perspectives are more frequent than ever. Healing Circles serve as a training ground for empathy, teaching individuals to appreciate the uniqueness of each person's journey while discovering the shared humanity that binds them together.

7.2 Overcoming Prejudice and Bias

Healing Circles provide a fertile ground to confront and overcome prejudice and bias. Chapter 7.2 explores how participants, within the context of a supportive and non-judgmental environment, confront and dismantle preconceived notions they may harbor about others. As they embrace empathy, they learn to embrace the richness that diverse perspectives offer.

In the face of current world challenges, such as social unrest and discrimination, Healing Circles become sanctuaries of inclusivity, challenging the barriers that divide us. Participants learn to recognize the common threads that weave us together, fostering a spirit of unity that transcends superficial differences.

7.3 Celebrating Differences and Shared Humanity

In Healing Circles, the celebration of differences goes hand in hand with recognizing shared humanity. Chapter 7.3 emphasizes how participants begin to see that, despite diverse experiences and backgrounds, they all share fundamental emotions and vulnerabilities. This shared humanity forms the foundation for building authentic connections and fostering deep empathy.

In the current world situation, marked by polarizing views and societal divides, Healing Circles stand as models of unity and understanding. Participants celebrate their differences while finding strength in the realization that, as human beings, they are intrinsically linked to one another.

Conclusion:
Chapter 7, "Embracing Diversity, Fostering Empathy," captures the essence of Healing Circles as crucibles of inclusivity and understanding. Within these transformative communities, participants learn to appreciate the beauty of diverse perspectives while embracing shared humanity. The celebration of differences and the cultivation of empathy offer profound healing potential, forging bonds of compassion that extend far beyond the confines of the therapy room.

In a world that grapples with divisiveness and discrimination, Healing Circles become beacons of hope, showing how embracing diversity can foster genuine connections and empower individuals to confront prejudice and bias. By nurturing empathy and understanding, these circles illuminate a path towards a more compassionate and united world, where the celebration of diversity becomes a catalyst for collective healing and growth.

–CHAPTER EIGHT–

The Art of Active Listening

In chapter 8 of "Healing Circles," we delve into the transformative art of active listening—a cornerstone of the therapeutic experience within these sacred spaces. Building on the power of storytelling that was explored in the initial contents of the book, this chapter illuminates how active listening becomes the catalyst for healing and connection among participants.

8.1 Deepening Communication within the Group

Healing Circles thrive on the principle of deep and meaningful communication. Chapter 8.1 emphasizes how active listening nurtures an atmosphere where participants feel genuinely heard and understood. As individuals share their stories, struggles, and triumphs, the art of active listening fosters a space where every voice is acknowledged with compassion and respect.

Just as Sara's journey in the initial storytelling section of the book showcased the transformative power of vulnerability and authentic storytelling, active listening becomes the canvas upon which her experiences are met with empathy. In the presence of compassionate peers, Sara's voice finds validation, inspiring her to explore her vulnerability even further and find solace in the collective wisdom of the group.

8.2 Developing Effective Listening Skills

Chapter 8.2 delves into the development of effective listening skills within Healing Circles. Participants learn to be fully present, setting aside distractions and judgments, to immerse themselves in the speaker's words. Through reflective listening and empathetic responses, individuals create an environment that encourages emotional exploration and healing.

In the context of Sarah's story, the women's empowerment group demonstrated how active listening becomes the bridge between participants' hearts. By honing their listening skills, group members validated Sarah's journey of self-discovery, enriching her sense of self-worth, and fostering an atmosphere of trust and vulnerability.

8.3 Providing Constructive Feedback and Support

Within the therapeutic sanctuary of Healing Circles, constructive feedback and support become vital components of active listening. Chapter 8.3 explores how participants offer gentle guidance and encouragement, empowering each other to confront challenges and embrace personal growth.

Mark's story of finding solace in a veterans' support group showcases the profound impact of constructive feedback and support. As the group actively listens to his experiences of war and post-traumatic stress, they offer non-judgmental feedback that allows Mark to navigate his emotional landscape with newfound clarity and resilience.

Conclusion:
Chapter 8, "The Art of Active Listening," celebrates the transformative power of truly hearing and understanding one another within Healing Circles. Through deep communication, effective listening skills, and constructive support, participants embrace the vulnerability of storytelling, creating a harmonious and empathetic therapeutic community.

HEALING CIRCLES

As participants share their stories and actively listen to one another, the healing threads of connection intertwine, weaving a tapestry of shared experiences and insights. The art of active listening enhances the profound impact of vulnerability and storytelling, fostering an environment where healing becomes a collective journey.

In a world that often prioritizes rapid communication and superficial interactions, Healing Circles stand as havens of deep and authentic connection. By mastering the art of active listening, participants kindle the embers of empathy, forging a path towards individual and collective healing that resonates beyond the confines of the group therapy setting.

–CHAPTER NINE–

Empowerment and Self-Discovery

In chapter 9 of "Healing Circles," we delve into the empowering journey of self-discovery that unfolds within these transformative therapeutic communities. Participants find themselves traversing the depths of their emotions, beliefs, and aspirations, unlocking the wellspring of strength within. This chapter explores how Healing Circles become catalysts for personal empowerment and self-awareness.

9.1 Unveiling the Layers of Self

Healing Circles provide a nurturing space for participants to peel away the layers of self, uncovering the essence of who they truly are. Chapter 9.1 delves into how the journey of self-discovery enables individuals to examine their past, confront their present, and envision their future.

Just as Daniel's story of confronting addiction within a group therapy setting revealed the power of vulnerability and peer support, the process of self-discovery becomes his compass. With the guidance of therapists and the empathy of peers, Daniel unveils the layers of his addiction, reclaiming the essence of his true self and igniting the flame of transformation.

9.2 Embracing Empowerment through Shared Growth

As participants embark on their transformative odyssey, they embrace the power of empowerment through shared growth. Chapter 9.2 highlights how the Healing Circles experience becomes a collective endeavor, where individuals celebrate one another's victories and lend support during moments of challenge.

In the context of Sarah's journey in the women's empowerment group, shared growth fosters a sense of sisterhood and collective empowerment. As each woman discovers her unique strengths and overcomes personal hurdles, the group finds inspiration in one another's triumphs, nurturing a profound sense of community and strength.

9.3 Discovering Resilience and Life Purpose

Within Healing Circles, individuals not only unearth resilience but also find a sense of life purpose. Chapter 9.3 delves into how confronting one's vulnerabilities and experiences of pain allows individuals to emerge with newfound strength and clarity of purpose.

HEALING CIRCLES

Drawing from Mark's story of finding solace in a veterans' support group, Healing Circles become incubators of resilience. Through the lens of shared experiences, Mark and his peers tap into a wellspring of courage, propelling them toward a sense of purpose beyond their past traumas.

How and Why:

The empowering journey of self-discovery within Healing Circles is fostered by a nurturing and empathetic environment. Participants are encouraged to explore their emotions, confront their vulnerabilities, and share their stories authentically.

The presence of skilled therapists and the compassionate support of peers form a strong foundation for personal growth and empowerment.

HEALING CIRCLES

The process of self-discovery unfolds through active listening, storytelling, and peer feedback. The collaborative setting of shared goals and the embrace of vulnerability create an atmosphere where individuals can explore their beliefs, values, and life experiences.

As participants connect with their authentic selves, they find the strength to transform pain into purpose and embrace their innate resilience.

In a world where external pressures and expectations can overshadow individual identity, Healing Circles become sanctuaries for self-exploration and growth. By empowering individuals to embrace their unique strengths and vulnerabilities, these therapeutic communities nurture self-awareness and lay the groundwork for a life imbued with purpose and authenticity.

HEALING CIRCLES

Within the tapestry of shared healing, participants find empowerment through the collective journey of self-discovery, leaving a lasting impact on their lives beyond the confines of the therapy room.

–CHAPTER TEN–

Beyond Healing Circles: Carrying the Torch of Transformation

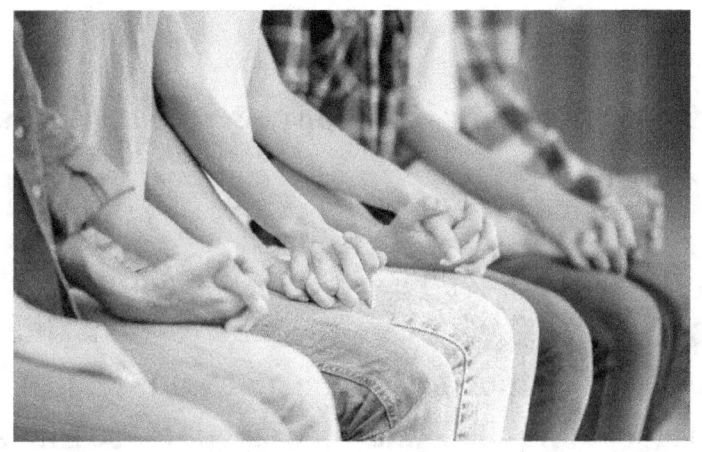

Chapter 10 of "Healing Circles" transcends the boundaries of the therapeutic space, exploring how the transformative power of these communities ripples outward, influencing the lives of participants beyond their time in the circle.

It delves into the concept of carrying the torch of transformation, illuminating how individuals become catalysts for positive change in their communities and the broader world.

10.1 Embracing the Journey of Continual Growth

In the final chapter of the book, participants in Healing Circles recognize that their journey of transformation does not end with the closing of the therapeutic sessions. Chapter 10.1 emphasizes how the empowering principles, insights, and connections forged within the circle become guiding lights in their ongoing quest for self-discovery and personal growth.

As individuals carry the torch of transformation, they remain open to continual learning and exploration. They acknowledge that life's challenges are ever-evolving, and healing is an ongoing process. Armed with newfound resilience and empathy, they navigate future obstacles with greater clarity and strength.

10.2 The Ripple Effect: Spreading Healing Beyond the Circle

The transformative impact of Healing Circles extends far beyond the individuals who participate. Chapter 10.2 explores the concept of the ripple effect—a phenomenon where the positive changes experienced within the group radiate outward, touching the lives of family, friends, and the community at large.

Empowered by their journey, participants become agents of positive change in their social circles.

They carry the wisdom of self-awareness, empathy, and active listening into their daily interactions, fostering deeper connections and inspiring others to embark on their healing journeys.

10.3 Advocating for Inclusivity and Mental Health Awareness

In the broader world, participants carry the torch of transformation as advocates for inclusivity and mental health awareness. Chapter 10.3 highlights how their experiences within Healing Circles galvanize them to break down societal stigmas and promote understanding and compassion.

Informed by their journey of embracing diversity and fostering empathy, individuals become passionate advocates for inclusivity, promoting spaces of acceptance and support for all. They use their stories and experiences to destigmatize mental health challenges and champion the importance of seeking help and support.

Conclusion:

Chapter 10, "Beyond Healing Circles: Carrying the Torch of Transformation," marks the culmination of the transformative journey experienced within these therapeutic communities. Participants understand that the healing and empowerment they found within the circle are not isolated events but stepping stones toward a lifelong path of growth and positive impact.

The ripple effect of Healing Circles extends beyond the confines of the therapeutic space, touching lives, and sparking change in families, communities, and society at large.

HEALING CIRCLES

By carrying the torch of transformation, participants become beacons of resilience, empathy, and advocacy—illuminating a path towards a world that embraces diversity, fosters understanding, and nurtures healing.

As Healing Circles participants step back into the broader world, they do so with a sense of purpose and a commitment to creating spaces of compassion and acceptance. Their collective journey of transformation inspires a ripple of positive change, leaving an indelible mark on the tapestry of humanity—one woven with threads of resilience, empathy, and the enduring power of healing.

–CHAPTER ELEVEN–

The Endless Circle of Gratitude

In the concluding chapter of "Healing Circles," we explore the profound significance of gratitude as the heartwarming thread that weaves together the transformative journey within these therapeutic communities.

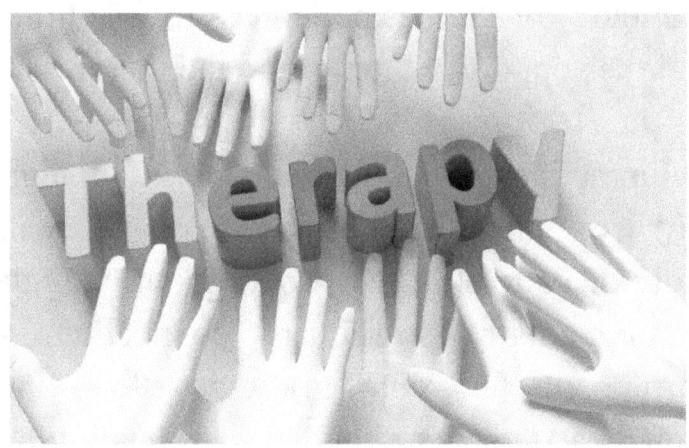

Chapter 11 delves into how the endless circle of gratitude forms a powerful loop of healing, connection, and personal growth.

11.1 Cultivating Gratitude as a Healing Practice

Healing Circles instill the practice of gratitude as a potent tool for healing and self-reflection. Chapter 11.1 emphasizes how participants are encouraged to express gratitude for their experiences, their journey, and the support of their peers and therapists.

The practice of gratitude becomes an integral part of the healing process, allowing individuals to shift their focus from struggles to moments of solace and connection. As participants cultivate gratitude, they open their hearts to the abundance of healing and positive change that Healing Circles have ushered into their lives.

11.2 Fostering a Sense of Connectedness

Within Healing Circles, the circle of gratitude fosters a profound sense of connectedness among participants. Chapter 11.2 explores how the practice of expressing gratitude for one another's support deepens the bonds within the group, forming an unbreakable thread of unity.

As individuals share their appreciation for the empathy, understanding, and kindness they have received from their peers, they forge connections that transcend the therapeutic space. The circle of gratitude becomes a conduit for love and support, empowering participants to continue uplifting one another long after the formal sessions have ended.

11.3 The Ripple Effect: Gratitude as a Force for Positive Change

Beyond the confines of the Healing Circles, gratitude extends its ripple effect into the broader world.

The practice of gratitude becomes a transformative force, influencing how individuals perceive the world and interact with others. Their expressions of thankfulness ripple outward, inspiring kindness, compassion, and empathy in those they encounter. As they continue to share the circle of gratitude, it enriches the lives of countless others, creating an endless loop of positivity and healing.

Conclusion:

"The Endless Circle of Gratitude," culminates the transformative journey within Healing Circles by illuminating the power of gratitude as a driving force of healing and positive change. The practice of gratitude becomes an integral part of the participants' lives, deepening connections and inspiring a ripple of kindness and empathy in the world.

The circle of gratitude nurtured within Healing Circles never truly ends. It perpetuates a timeless cycle of healing and connection, uniting individuals in their shared experiences of growth and resilience. The unbroken thread of gratitude continues to weave its way through the tapestry of human connections, reminding us of the profound impact that healing communities can have on the human spirit.